MW01101033

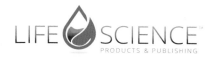

Copyright © 2018 Life Science Publishing with Star Moree and Kari McDermott
1.800.336.6308, www.DiscoverLSP.com
Printed in the United States of America 10 9 8 7 6 5 4 3 2 1

All rights reserved. No part of this book may be reproduced or transmitted in any form or by any means, electronic or mechanical, including photocopying, recording, or by any information storage and retrieval system, without permission in writing from the author(s) and publisher.

Life Science Publishing is the publisher of this book and is not responsible for its content. The information contained herein is for educational purposes only and as a guideline for your personal use. It should not be used as a substitute for medical counseling with a health professional. The author(s) and publisher are not rendering professional advice or services. The author(s) shall have neither liability nor responsibility to any person or entity with respect to any loss or damage caused, or alleged to have been caused, directly or indirectly by the information or recipes in this book. The author(s) and publisher do not accept responsibility for such use.

Although the author(s) have made every effort to ensure the accuracy of the information contained in this book, we assume no responsibility for errors or omissions.

Neither the author(s) nor the publisher advocate the use of any other essential oils without Young Living Essential Oils, LC's exclusive Seed to Seal® guarantee. Even minor changes in the quality of an essential oil may render it, at best, useless and, at worst, dangerous. The use of essential oils should be done with thorough study, watchful care, and judicious prudence.

Content adapted from:

    Beat the Blues DIY: Keys to Wellness ©2017

Used with permission of publisher *Essentials for Healthy Living, Inc.*, and authors Star Moree and Kari McDermott.

FOREWORD

Star Moree and Kari McDermott are pioneers in Young Living and lead the way with a collection of education that teaches simple and effective tips on using essential oils and products. Their work has been respected for its ability to create fun and useful Make-And-Take products that attract new oil users. It is a perfect way to share the oils and teach people how to live without harsh chemicals.

Once again, the duo has created a volume that teaches you about improving your mood! Our emotions affect everything we do – our communication, productivity, relationships, and health. Many times, we neglect this area of our lives and just keep pushing forward in this relentless 24/7 world. That is always a mistake—one that so many of us find ourselves making as we strive to do our best. In order to have true wellness and good health, our mood matters just as much as our physical health.

It begins with what we eat, where we spend our time, how much water we drink and so much more. This book gives us guidance for each area of our lives we need to focus on to improve our feelings and moods—which in turn, helps to improve our overall physical health. These are wonderful tips and ideas on the simple things we can do each day that help to improve our feelings.

I know from personal experience the difference I have felt and experienced when I have incorporated these recommendations in my life. My outlook is more positive and that becomes contagious to everyone around me. Positive feelings equal positive results. Educating people with these simple truths can be so life changing!

I invite you to educate yourself and others using the information contained in this volume. Young Living's unique oils and products truly work. Sharing these products and these truths with others helps to improve the wellness of the ones we love. It is truly fulfilling when you see others benefit in such a positive way from products that are healthy and chemical-free. It helps to fulfill the mission of spreading Young Living Essential Oils to every home in the world.

May you use this information to discover greater joy, greater health, and greater abundance in your life!

Love. Learn. Share.

xoxo

Troie Battles

Troie Storms-Battles

AUTHOR MESSAGE

As a Young Living member since 1998, thankfully, I've had the privilege of raising my family within a household of essential oils.

I have supported both our daughter and our son in very competitive year-round sports (figure skating and hockey) and in being good students—both in school and at home. These oils are a true "Gift from God" that I believe offer them the "competitive edge" along with improving their ability to learn, focus, and maintain their creative talents.

Searching for the best products for our family, friends and clients led us to Young Living Essential Oils. We have aligned with Young Living because the company holds itself to the seed to seal standard we were looking for— to create healthier people and a healthier planet.

One of the things that I appreciated so much about being involved with Young Living is that we not only found a Wellness Company, we found a Wellness Community. While Young Living provides the highest quality essential oils and nutritional products, there is also the mindfulness of caring for the earth and each other! It is a community of like-minded people that are interested in looking at all aspects of our wellness, based on problem solving and raising awareness.

This booklet touches on many of the issues we as humans face on a daily basis to stay above the Wellness line. By combining essential oils, the power of nutrition, clean water, fresh air and other highlights we've shared, we can "Beat the Blues" and enjoy the best that life has to offer.

We invite you to share our passion to provide Education and help create a world filled with Wellness, Purpose, and Abundance.

Sincerely,

Star Moree

AUTHOR MESSAGE

More and more people are seeking "Wellness." And more and more evidence has come to light that it is based on lifestyle choices! Sixteen years ago, I aligned with "a Star" and a company that shared my values. I love the sun, the water, fresh air, earth's beauty, garden bounty and all the resources that nature reveals to me. I knew that surrounding myself with smart, mindful people, guaranteed my journey on a whole-life-wellness path, rather than accepting that life creates dis-ease and there's a pill for that.

For me, wellness comes from observing nature's balance and the decisions we make, based on that knowledge and current research. We know sugar is addictive, toxins are harmful, that we need sleep, water, sun, minerals and fresh fruits and vegetables to support our bodies.

It doesn't matter where your knowledge base is right now. This little book might be the first simple tool you've ever used or it might be an opportunity to show other people some basic tips to help them 'stay above the wellness line.' We love supporting Young Living members, students, teachers, leaders and followers of the wellness industry and.... Thank God.... the shifting paradigm!

It is our desire and our intention to help people create a life filled with Wellness, full of Purpose and feeling Abundant on their personal journeys. Just remember, the journey never ends, it just expands and evolves. Through our authorship and relationship with Young Living and the Life Science Publishing staff, we want everyone to reach their Highest Potential.... and we know you can't get there without good health!

I hope you find some useful keys in this book to apply to your Do It Yourself Wellness journey.

Sincerely,

Kari McDermott

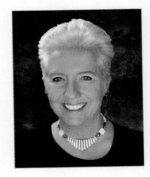

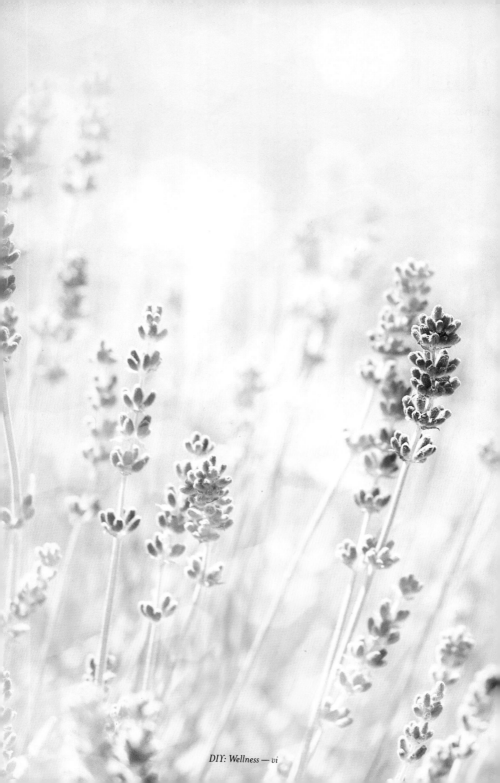

TABLE OF CONTENTS

BRING THE OUTDOORS IN

Our disconnect from nature is a disconnect to our "life source," our spirit, emotions and to each other. When our deepest desires or greatest fears seem overwhelming and we do not take a deep breath or move our body, the lack of action keeps our thoughts stagnant. Action is the key to shifting a negative or stuck emotion.... and getting outside, is a FREE remedy for change!

Going outside, taking a walk, choosing any physical activity that requires you to be outdoors will naturally uplift your spirit and set fresh, new thoughts in motion. Even rain and snow, not just sun and flowers, effect your sense of smell, sight, sound, touch, and confidence. Every element of an outdoor environment has qualities that we innately tune into that release endorphins and organize the chatter in our heads.

Think about a vision or dream that seems out of reach from the couch, your bed, your office, or your repetitive thoughts. Visions stay stuck wherever you're thoughts are stuck! You have to take action. If you constantly try to pursue your goals from a pattern that isn't working, you have to change the environment you are in. Movement is absolutely required to shift stagnant thought patterns into active energy!

Every season and even cycles of the moon can influence our moods. A bouquet of flowers, a bowl of fruit, the scent of a seasonal meal (especially out of season), and the scent of any plant effects us. Aromas captured in our minds, can unlock memories in our hearts, soften the feelings of despair and shift our emotions toward safety and success.

Even for a brief moment, diffusing and inhaling essential oils is the cheapest, fastest method of triggering a positive, chemical reaction in your brain than anything we can think of..... if and when we can't go outside and surround ourselves with nature's scents and Mother Earth's free remedies.

If you can't be outdoors, then bring the outdoors in.

Unlock and open the door with the following keys!

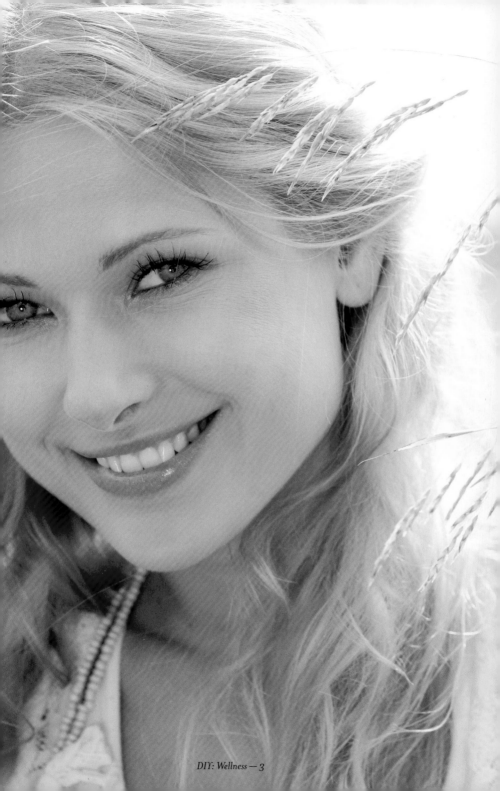

THE POWER OF ESSENTIAL OILS

Aromatherapy has a long history and its place in wellness programs has finally overpowered the skeptics. If you still come across one, offer them a drop of Frankincense to lighten their spirit. Tell them you're on a journey to beat the blues without them!

Even before a drop of oil reaches the palm of your hand, it has left a complex, molecular code in the air. Within seconds, each molecule connects to your brain. We were, are, and will always be, connected to the essence of the plant kingdom. This has never changed. It's just been forgotten. Earth was a plant kingdom first. Plants set the tone, and can survive without us, but we won't survive without them. Maybe we owe them some respect and gratitude.

It's time to reduce toxic chemicals in exchange for the scented, natural kingdom we were born into. There's an intelligence that may seem beyond our scope, but it's actually available in every drop of essential oil.

Experience is the best teacher! The more you choose an oil for emotional shifts, changes in attitude, or to reduce physical stress.... the faster you will see some results. Citrus oils might be your first option to freshen a beverage or brighten your day. They truly carry sunshine and rainbows in every drop!

Other great beginnings:
- lavender to soothe your sun-kissed skin
- peppermint to cool your feet and sharpen your mind
- tea tree oil for seasonal pests

Don't expose skin to UV rays for 24 to 48 hours after applying when using citrus essential oils. Learn about the various types to protect skin sensitivity. Wise use of essential oils will increase your results and minimize any unnecessary negative reactions.

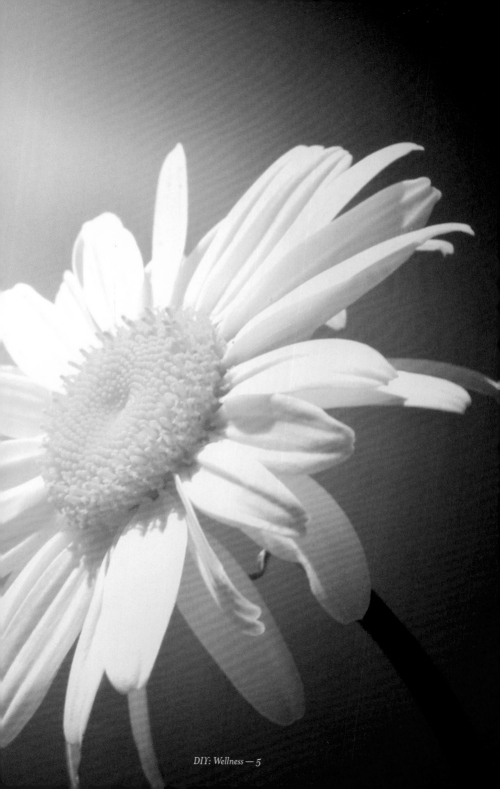

JUST BREATHE

We are all related! We all breathe!

"The Butterfly Effect" says everything we do to the planet, we do to ourselves and future generations. Our grandchildren will breathe the air we pollute. They will drink the water we poison. They will eat the food we contaminate or they will thrive by our choices to protect the elements that give us life. Spreading the message about essential oils seems like a good way to build healthier, more connected relationships.

Most of us have about 30 seconds of life left when oxygen is compromised. Basic biology taught us that trees and plants convert carbon dioxide into oxygen. Our lives depend on plants and we know that constant, low oxygen at a cellular level, creates illness and disease. Did you know that essential oils raise your oxygen levels –just like plants!

What a beautiful and simple way to breathe deeper, fill your lungs, smell the essence of life, and expand your own horizons! Menthol, pine, and eucalyptus oils open our sinuses and lungs so they are perfect for lifting any cloudy moods or 'overcast' feelings!

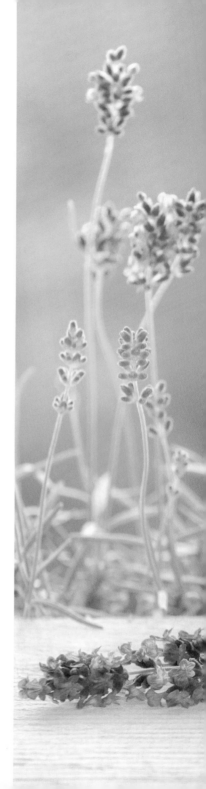

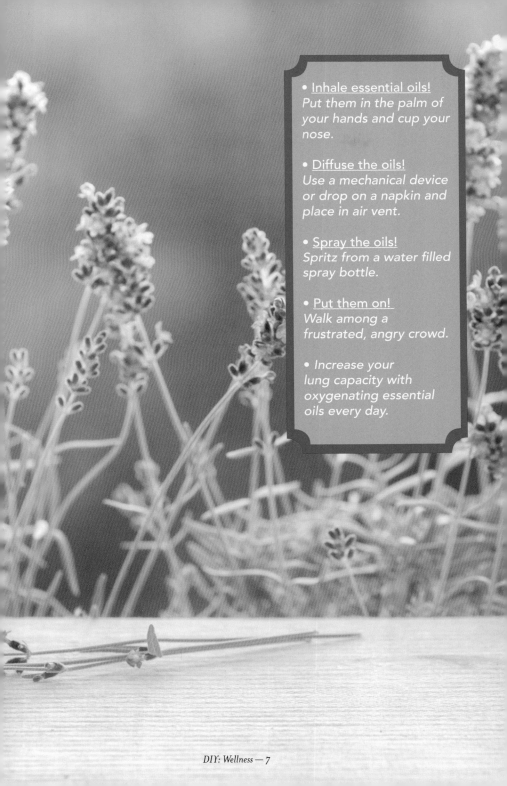

- <u>Inhale essential oils!</u> *Put them in the palm of your hands and cup your nose.*

- <u>Diffuse the oils!</u> *Use a mechanical device or drop on a napkin and place in air vent.*

- <u>Spray the oils!</u> *Spritz from a water filled spray bottle.*

- <u>Put them on!</u> *Walk among a frustrated, angry crowd.*

- *Increase your lung capacity with oxygenating essential oils every day.*

THE POWER OF THE SUN

- Every essential oil carries the Power of the Sun... open the bottle and let it out.

- Citrus Oils make a great food and beverage additive.

- Inhale, Diffuse or apply to bottom of feet (UV sensitive).

- Make a Light Box to increase happiness.

- Change lightbulbs to LED natural tone.

- Stay away from the Sick American Diet.

- Supplement with vitamin D3 and 5-HTP.

For decades we have been told to be afraid of the sun. Why? Isn't the sun a life-giving, primary source to our existence here on earth?

Does our fear have evidence-based science to warrant never going outdoors? Do we listen to one-sided views? Have you read the scientific studies on the chemical ingredients in sunscreen or any of the millions of toxic products introduced over the last six decades that we breathe, smear on our skin, and ingest?

The sun is not the cause of our ill-health. We are! It's time for people to use some common sense, instead of relying on products that are harmful to our health. Honor the sun a little more, and advertising a lot less.

If you can, use full spectrum light bulbs, reduce 'blue-screen-time' and supplement the sun's relationship to our lives with D3 and vitamin K. Every essential oil carries chemical traits from its environment, so the sun is part of every drop!

**Note: There's a Rainbow hidden in ....
Every Drop of Essential Oil!**

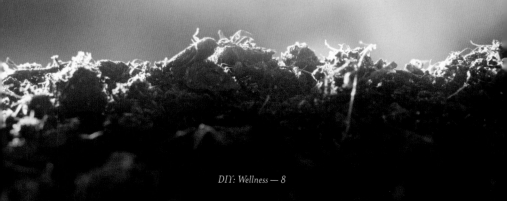

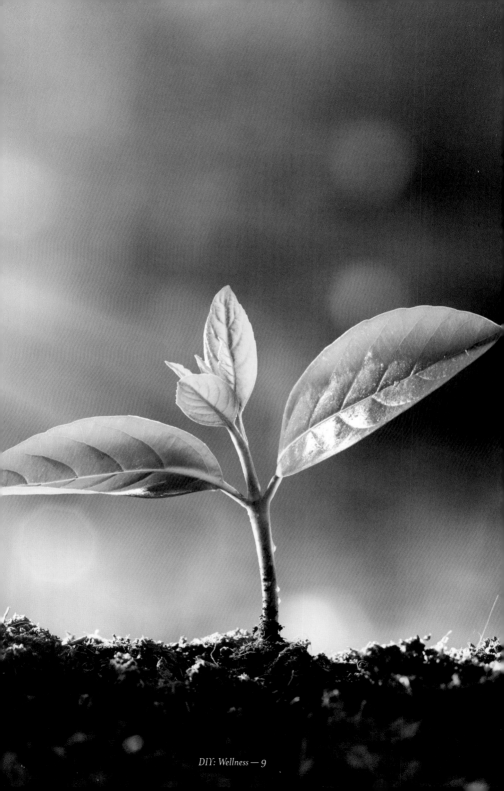

WATER IS LIFE

We are approximately 65% water.

Our brains are 73% water! Shouldn't our intelligence absorb that fact? The earth is 71% water. We come from a warm pool of water in our mother's womb. Why would we forget to hold that sacred or feel indifferent about it?

The importance of water is second only to oxygen. It is a basic necessity to all life. It shouldn't be controlled, owned, or destroyed by one group of people over the birth rights of another. We were all given this key!

There is no substitute for water! Anything you put in water alters its purity to flush your digestive system (except an essential oil). Fluoride, chlorine, and bromine can be added to water, but they are not one of the 12 minerals our bodies need. Read up on iodine and ask why it is used in remote areas to purify water, but not in our municipal water sources?

Alcohol, soda pop, and sugary drinks are detrimental to the liver and kidneys and your brain power. Minimize the use of 'fake drinks' to quench your thirst. (Try "Sole Water" recipe to start your day.)

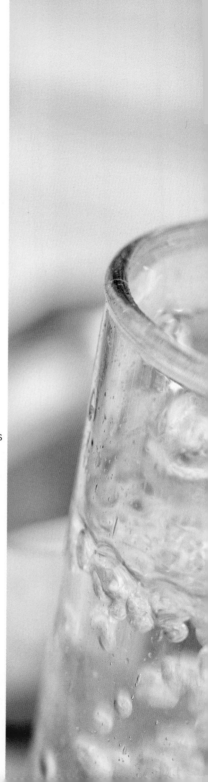

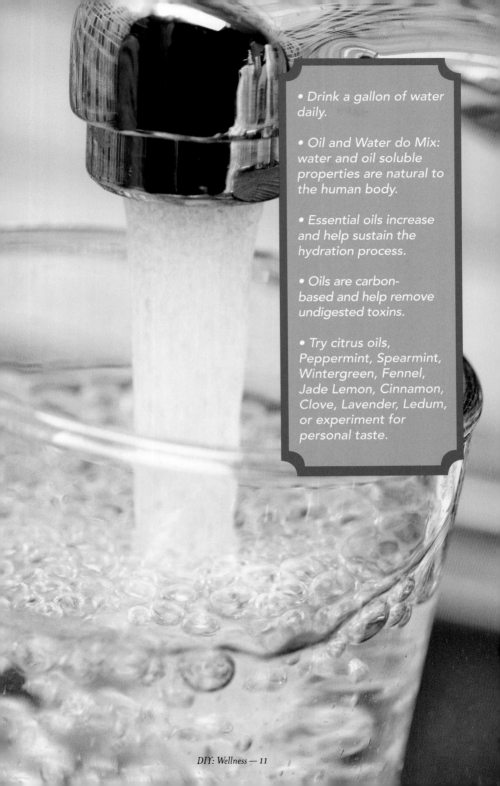

• Drink a gallon of water daily.

• Oil and Water do Mix: water and oil soluble properties are natural to the human body.

• Essential oils increase and help sustain the hydration process.

• Oils are carbon-based and help remove undigested toxins.

• Try citrus oils, Peppermint, Spearmint, Wintergreen, Fennel, Jade Lemon, Cinnamon, Clove, Lavender, Ledum, or experiment for personal taste.

THE POWER OF NUTRITION

We need proteins, carbohydrates, and fats. Each has to be 'assimilated' in order to be converted into energy to sustain our health. Nutrition should be a primary part of education from kindergarten to medical school. "Food Science" may be complicated under academic disciplines, but from soil to seed– to how it nourishes our bodies, it's really not that hard!

The Food Pyramid has changed many times as we discover new insights about nutrition as a foundation for wellness, and to prevent disease. Vegetables and fruits have finally been recognized as the basis of good health, at the base of the pyramid.

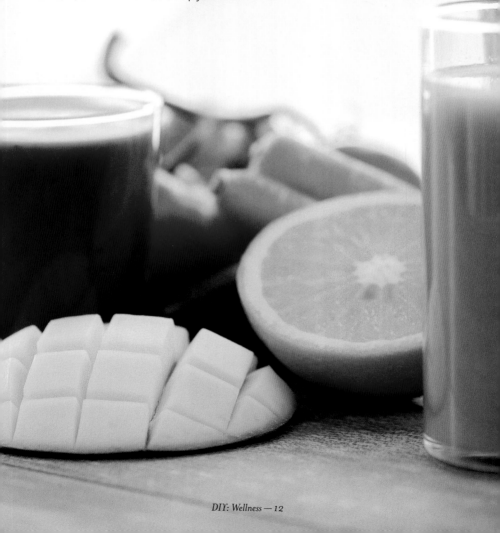

Whole grains and plant oils are second. Legumes, nuts, and seeds are third. Eggs, fish, poultry, and plant proteins are fourth. Meat proteins, including dairy, soy, and red meat, are best eaten at a minimum. Sugar and processed 'foods' are at the top of the pyramid (0-1 serving).

Essential oils aren't 'nutrients,' but are partners in the breakdown of nutrients to support the body's ability to absorb what it needs and eliminate what it doesn't.

- *Increase the volume of fresh, organic vegetables and fruits you eat.*

- *Get a blender, food processor or juicer and concentrate the nutrients.*

- *Make smoothies that taste good and supply you with daily vitamins and minerals.*

- *Wash store-bought produce with Lemon or other citrus oils.*

- *Keep Essential Oils on the spice rack, in the kitchen. (Use sparingly – with a toothpick to start.)*

YOU ARE WHAT YOU EAT

So don't be fast, cheap, easy or fake!

The "New Science" is just restating what Adele Davis wrote about over sixty years ago. Maybe it's not so "new." There is more than enough proof to suggest our eating habits have caused a lot of problems and we need to get back to a healthy diet in order to thrive and return to vibrant energy required for clear thinking, happiness, and longevity!

Plants absorb "the light" of the photosynthesis process. Essential oils retain "the light" and are 100x to 1,000x more potent than foods and herbs! Adding healthy, pure essential oils to your food and beverages is easy!

Everything is Energy! Vitamins and minerals equate to levels of 'real energy.' Your thoughts and actions are energy! Your brain and digestive system are linked to the messages you send: "I LOVE MY BODY and MY LIFE!"

You can find lists of the important vitamins and minerals a body needs, but You have to experiment.... and You have to tune into Your Body! Include Amino acids; B complex; C/D E; Enzymes/Probiotic; Minerals; Fibers; Good Fats, and a Rainbow of Food.

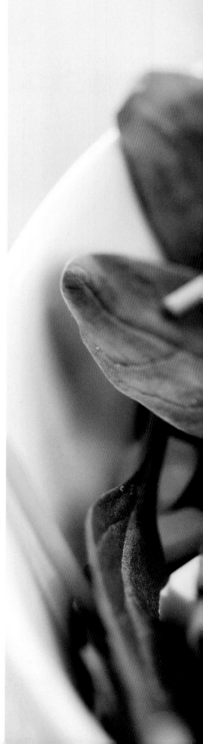

Top 10 Foods to AVOID

• Microwave popcorn

• Fat-free ice cream

• Sugar substitutes & artificial sweeteners

• Canned soup

• Big Ag Fruits: apples, strawberries, grapes, peaches & nectarines

• Big Ag corn is GMO used in all processed foods and fed to animals

• Margarine = trans fats, hydrogenated

• Hot dogs, bacon, cold cuts, cured meats

• Donuts = sugar, GMO (flour, corn, soy-fillers), unhealthy fats

• Swordfish is highest in mercury content

THE POWER OF MOVEMENT

- *Apply essential oils before and after exercise.*

- *Set a cell memory pattern by applying them every day.*

- *Create an EO ritual for the mind, body & spirit.*

- *Connect your breath and thoughts to your body with EOs.*

- *Enhance flexibility and reduce tension in joints & muscles.*

- *Joints & muscles love conifer trees, menthol-based, herb varieties and blends.*

Age and health will determine what form of movements we can take, starting with a baby's natural reflexes and ending with a final heart beat and last breath. In between, our body relies on our ability to move, flex and stretch to build resilience over a long period of time. If we don't or we can't, there will be consequences to our well-being at various times in our lives, affecting the length and quality of it.

Every organ and body system requires movement. Stagnation and atrophy decrease the size of our muscles, organs and tissue, which restricts the flow of blood and other fluids. So, even if you have a setback to your health, the sooner you start moving again, the better!

Essential oils actually have chemical compounds that stimulate the brain to a more positive state of mind, and a positive state of mind motivates us to movement and recovery. Inhaling or diffusing can be the first step to activity and many more days of a vibrant existence. Remember to "bring the outdoors in" to stimulate a fast return to physical health.

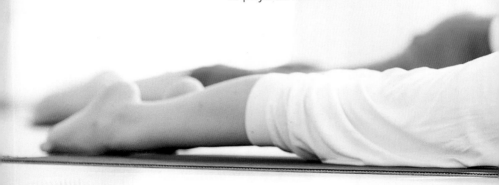

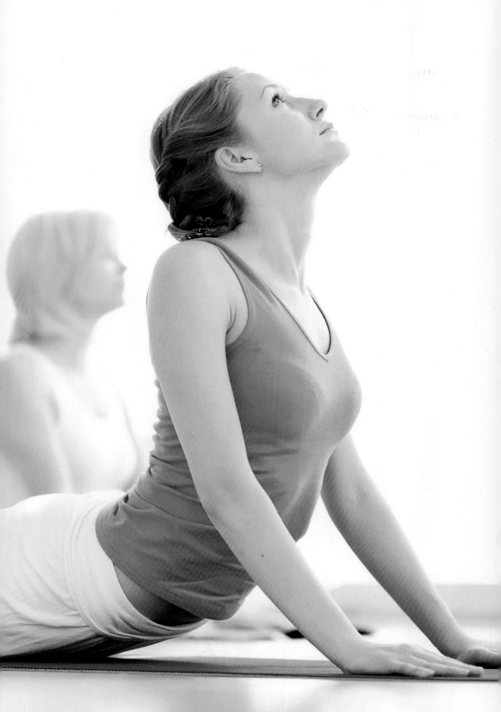

THE EMOTIONAL CELL

Few people think about their health at a cellular level, but it is the core and code of life. Our bodies are amazing at repairing themselves given the right tools. Since our emotions are tied to our will to live, it's important that there's someone around who cares! We respond to love and community at a cellular level. Cells hold "memories" of every interaction.

Cell health is about keeping things in balance. We are actually made up of more bacteria than cells. And the evidence of the mitochondria that creates the energy, fuels every action, and empowers proper cell function makes cell health a foundational piece to life. The mitochondria also help form, decompose and remove 'bad codes' from our DNA, which helps balance our hormones. This is an exciting branch of science that includes epigenetics. Our cells are listening!

- Healthy relationships have been proven to support our immune system.
- Staying connected keeps us vital and happy.
- Being touched stimulates the brain to produce "feel good chemicals."
- Pleasure is an emotion and cells remember how we treat each other.
- 12 hugs a day for cell maintenance.

Don't forget that Antioxidants are key to fighting free radicals and reducing the occurrences of inflammation and damaged cells. Whole Foods and Super Foods will prove their worth at a cellular level. Start young with super foods for your super powers to develop!

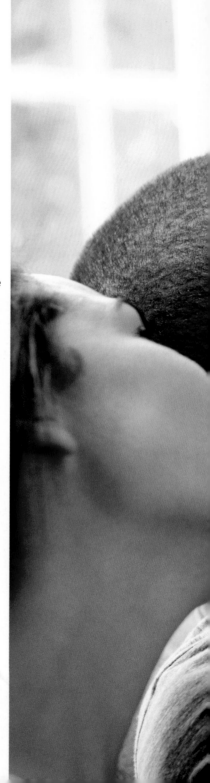

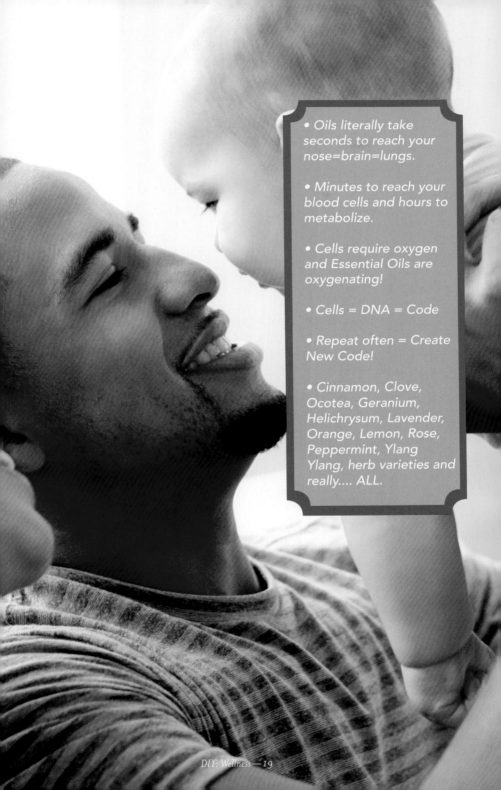

- Oils literally take seconds to reach your nose=brain=lungs.

- Minutes to reach your blood cells and hours to metabolize.

- Cells require oxygen and Essential Oils are oxygenating!

- Cells = DNA = Code

- Repeat often = Create New Code!

- Cinnamon, Clove, Ocotea, Geranium, Helichrysum, Lavender, Orange, Lemon, Rose, Peppermint, Ylang Ylang, herb varieties and really.... ALL.

THE POWER OF SLEEP

Have you ever heard the saying that you "heal while you sleep?"

Rejuvenation requires a state of rest for the body to repair. That's why sleep is so critical to our daily replenishment of energy at the cellular level and to reduce mental stress.

Lack of rest and sleep creates stress and acid in the system, which creates inflammation and imbalance in the microbiome (gut flora).

Research has proven that a lack of sleep can lead to serious health problems, decreased productivity, poor memory, weight gain, and critical thought processes. Sleep deprivation increases the risk for more serious conditions including depression, substance abuse, diabetes, and auto-immune disease. It also inhibits recovery from any injuries, pain, trauma, and major illness. Without sleep, our resistance to viruses, bacteria and even parasites can give them the upper hand.

Beauty can be 'skin deep' and we can usually spot the weary, tired, sleep deprived people we work, study, or share a life with!

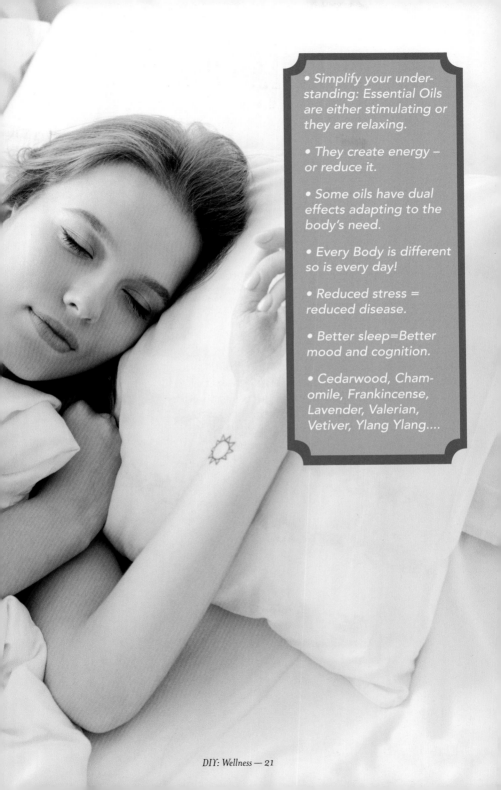

- Simplify your understanding: Essential Oils are either stimulating or they are relaxing.

- They create energy – or reduce it.

- Some oils have dual effects adapting to the body's need.

- Every Body is different so is every day!

- Reduced stress = reduced disease.

- Better sleep=Better mood and cognition.

- Cedarwood, Chamomile, Frankincense, Lavender, Valerian, Vetiver, Ylang Ylang....

THE HORMONE CONNECTION

The Endocrine System is being attacked by every "hormone disrupter" man has created. That includes fake food, packaging, clothing, bedding, furniture, carpet, most building materials, and every source of electrical power that makes life seem easy, with a flick of a switch.

Each generation continues to see a decrease in hormonal balance, thyroid function, diabetes, and adrenal fatigue. This is the path of the glandular system that starts with the pituitary, delivers hormones and then relies on the thyroid, pancreas, and adrenals to participate in a failing system. Age can diminish some of these functions, but modern lifestyle choices are the primary culprit.

Plants have a reproductive system, too! They are uniquely qualified to support us and stimulate our body systems safely. This science isn't new, it's just becoming more prevalent out of necessity to address our endocrine imbalances: low hormone levels, infertility, miscarriage, and heartache. It's not about the 'birds and the bees" ....it's about plants!

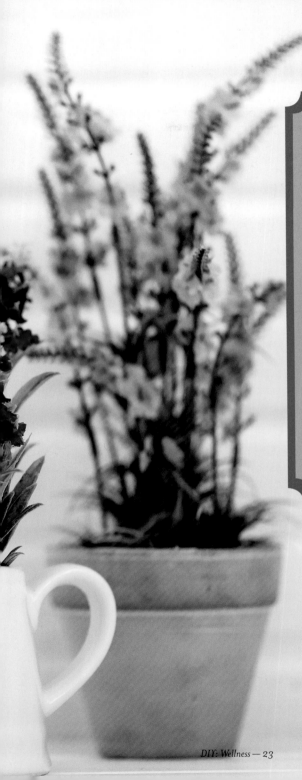

- Plants hold intelligence for reproduction and life cycles.

- Essential Oils carry a reproductive code from a viable seed.

- We have contaminated our world.

- The Endocrine System is God's channel for "our light."

- Chemicals disrupt the endocrine system. Nature supports it.

- Reduce EMFs.

- Angelica, Bergamot, Clary Sage, Lavender, Frankincense, Myrrh, Myrtle, Ylang Ylang....

METABOLISM POWER

- *Our ability to metabolize chemically grown, poisoned and processed foods is effecting our thyroid.*

- *The thyroid regulates our energy, our hormones and our future!*

- *Depletion of vitamins & minerals is a depletion of life.*

- *Essential Oil can curb or stimulate appetite.*

- *Clary Sage, Ylang Ylang, Blue Spruce, Geranium, Peppermint, Jasmine, Fennel, Angelica....*

This critical function is regulated by your thyroid and your digestive health. It's hard to say which is more important. If you have been exposed to too many products that have hormone disrupters, your thyroid function will diminish. If your diet contains too many processed foods, GMOs, sugar and bad fats, your digestive path will lead to mental fatigue.

It's all relative! A slow metabolism can be the direct result of imbalanced hormones that are regulated by the entire endocrine system. Isolating the thyroid, 'as the only cause for fatigue' is not the best advice. Poor digestive health leads to malabsorption of vitamins and minerals and the inability to eliminate toxins. These are key elements of the potential energy a better lifestyle will give you.

Be assertive when talking to your healthcare professional about fatigue. Be educated on the Endocrine System as a whole. It could save you years of guessing games and piles of money!

Follow the path of the pituitary, hypothalamus, thyroid/parathyroid, adrenal glands, pancreas, ovaries, and testis to see how our biology is impacted by our lifestyle choices.

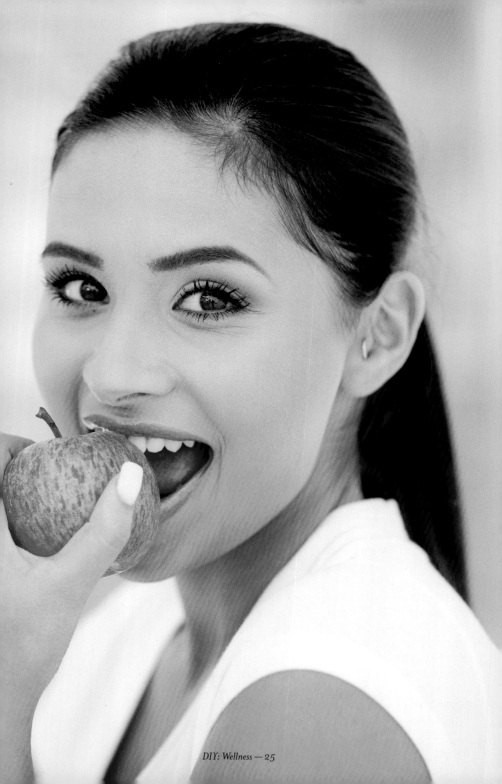

IODINE ON THE TABLE

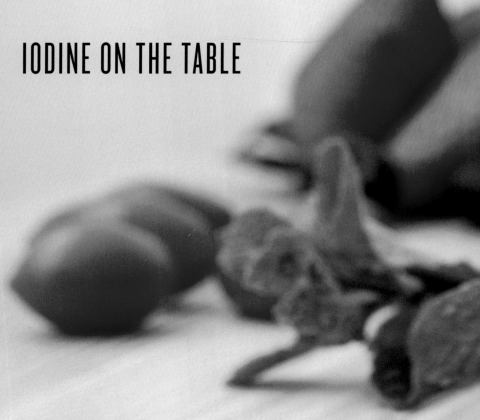

Iodine is directly related to the endocrine system. It supports our thyroid function, hormonal health, adrenal glands.... and stress. A resurgence of evidence to include iodine in our diets might make our vitamins and minerals more viable.

Iodine was demonized along with coconut oil, hemp and many other natural remedies during the evolution of pharmaceutical drugs, chemical fertilizers, pesticides in agriculture, and synthetic products. Who determines "what is best – through science?" Academia, that was once objective –or corporations marketing products using "science," as if it was objective, but is now "corrupted science."

Fluorine, bromine, and chlorine deplete our bodies of iodine every day. Most municipal water systems have "safe levels" determined by a branch of science that refuses to embrace new evidence put before them. Biased science, based on profits, has created huge divisions of trust, confusion, and health care advice.

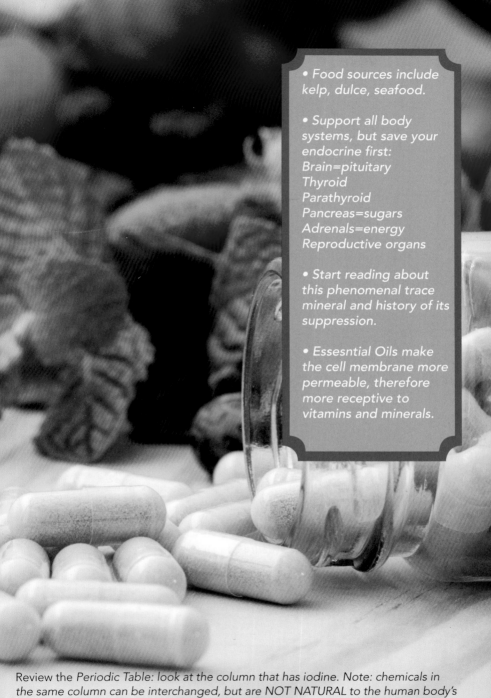

- Food sources include kelp, dulce, seafood.

- Support all body systems, but save your endocrine first:
Brain=pituitary
Thyroid
Parathyroid
Pancreas=sugars
Adrenals=energy
Reproductive organs

- Start reading about this phenomenal trace mineral and history of its suppression.

- Essesntial Oils make the cell membrane more permeable, therefore more receptive to vitamins and minerals.

Review the *Periodic Table:* look at the column that has iodine. Note: chemicals in the same column can be interchanged, but are NOT NATURAL to the human body's microbiome. Iodine is the only natural mineral in the column, yet fluorine, chlorine and bromine are used interchangeably and extensively, but have proven harmful to our health.

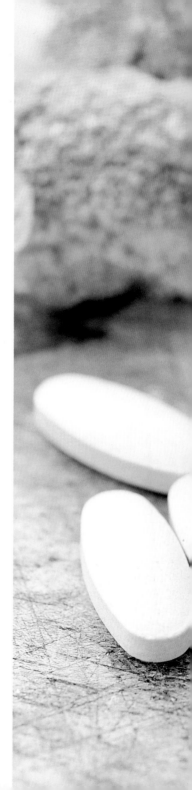

THE POWER OF MINERALS

We forget that we are made up of the substances of the earth! We are sun, water, air, soil, minerals, seed, food, virus, bacteria, and parasites all living together. We are a living biome. While we spend community time and intelligence seeking "the balance in nature," we need to spend just as much time looking at ourselves as living beings, with depleted resources that are out of balance.

Minerals that have been depleted from our soil, are depleted in our food, therefore they are depleted from our bodies at a cellular level. The five major minerals in the human body are calcium, phosphorus, magnesium, potassium, and sodium. Trace minerals include iodine, iron, cobalt, copper, zinc, manganese, molybdenum, and selenium.

Without a healthy supply of minerals we decrease the assimilation of water, vitamins and other nutrients. Magnesium and calcium are known to help us relax and thus repair. Two primary trace minerals getting more notice for their power to revitalize us, are iodine and iron.

Minerals are key.... to both our restful nights and daily energy levels!

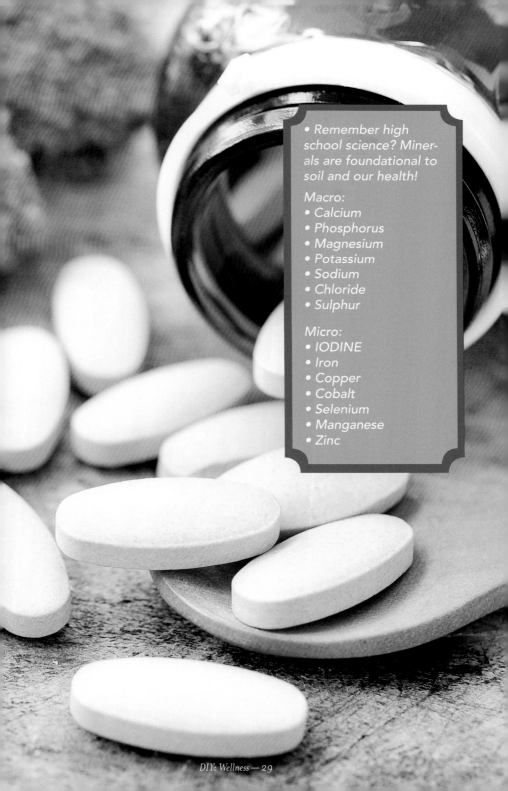

• Remember high school science? Minerals are foundational to soil and our health!

Macro:
- *Calcium*
- *Phosphorus*
- *Magnesium*
- *Potassium*
- *Sodium*
- *Chloride*
- *Sulphur*

Micro:
- *IODINE*
- *Iron*
- *Copper*
- *Cobalt*
- *Selenium*
- *Manganese*
- *Zinc*

GOOD FAT, BAD FAT

Reducing and even eliminating 'fat,' has proven to be bad advice. Heart disease increased over the decades, following the 'diet experts' advice. Experts are sometimes spokespeople for industry-based and biased science, so it usually takes a few decades to see the real results or consequences.

The proof is pretty clear about transfats and their association with processed foods that are doing so much harm. When whole foods are stripped of their value, fat, sugar and salt are added to make them taste good again.

Coconut oil was demonized by an industry that didn't want the competition. Crisco and margarine were touted as better for you than butter. Soy, canola, and corn are easy to grow, harvest and preserve so, they can be added to everything. History tends to bend favors for an industry, often at the expense of our health and our future.

Corporate farming is secured by lobbyists, subsidies, and by the media as a "safe promise" to the public that they're "feeding the world." Real food and real health doesn't come from the Big-Ag-Industry!

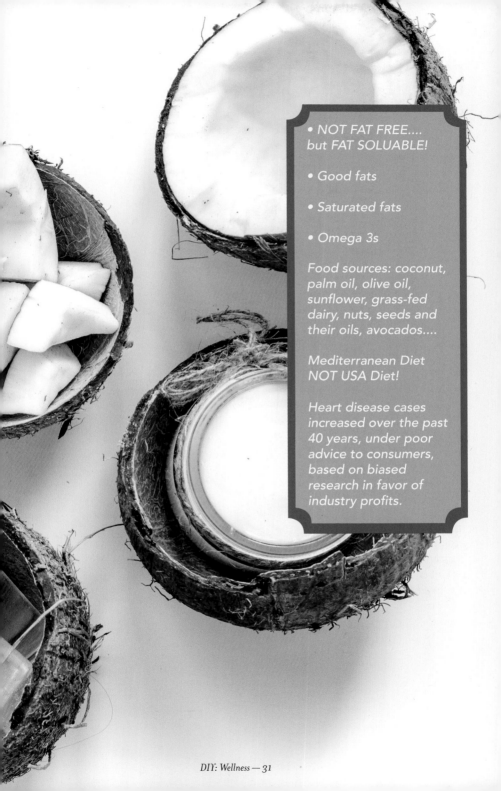

- NOT FAT FREE.... but FAT SOLUABLE!

- Good fats

- Saturated fats

- Omega 3s

Food sources: coconut, palm oil, olive oil, sunflower, grass-fed dairy, nuts, seeds and their oils, avocados....

Mediterranean Diet NOT USA Diet!

Heart disease cases increased over the past 40 years, under poor advice to consumers, based on biased research in favor of industry profits.

ENZYMES AND 5-HTP

Brain food! Who wouldn't like to improve the clarity of their thoughts or reduce the feelings of being overwhelmed? Enzymes are key to the digestive system. They break down our food and are critical to our brain's responses. "Did I receive the nutrients necessary to think? Did I assimilate the fats, carbohydrates, and proteins to satisfy my hungry brain?"

There is substantial research on how our brain works and the harm that synthetic medications can have on our ability to think clearly and live happy, healthy lives. As we become better informed and educated about the long term side effects of synthetic medication, the potential for 'real' food-based habits and natural supplementation, we'll reduce the damage to our overall health, pocket books, and realize our potential genius!

5-HTP has become a popular dietary supplement, because our food values have diminished. It is an essential amino acid and a key player as a building block for proteins that you get from 'real' food. And remember.... the Brain Loves Proteins!

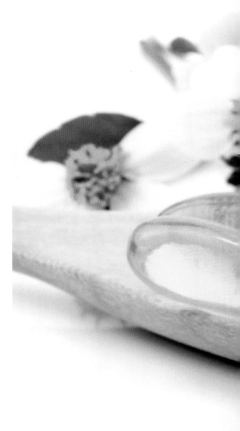

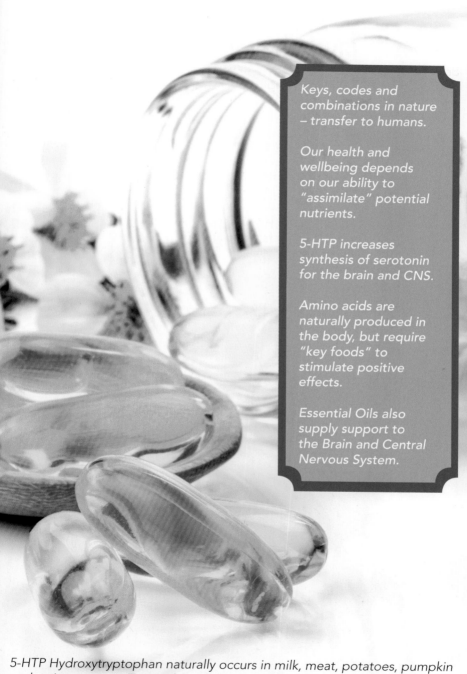

Keys, codes and combinations in nature – transfer to humans.

Our health and wellbeing depends on our ability to "assimilate" potential nutrients.

5-HTP increases synthesis of serotonin for the brain and CNS.

Amino acids are naturally produced in the body, but require "key foods" to stimulate positive effects.

Essential Oils also supply support to the Brain and Central Nervous System.

5-HTP Hydroxytryptophan naturally occurs in milk, meat, potatoes, pumpkin and various greens. Tryptophan alone may be an alternative for sensitive digestive systems.

A GREEN LEAFY WORLD

Have you ever noticed that most of the earth is green with vegetation and blue with water? When you get close to a garden of flowers or vegetables, every color of the rainbow comes into play. When you stand back and take in the big picture, life is a rainbow with a big green center!

If we could integrate these natural occurrences of color into how we eat and live, we could spend more time enjoying our affinity to a green world and less time being tired, crabby, overweight, sick and dying of our colorless, fake food and bad choices.

It's a choice, not a hunt for someone or something to blame. Enough of us have better answers and can play a role in educating others about "where most disease comes from."

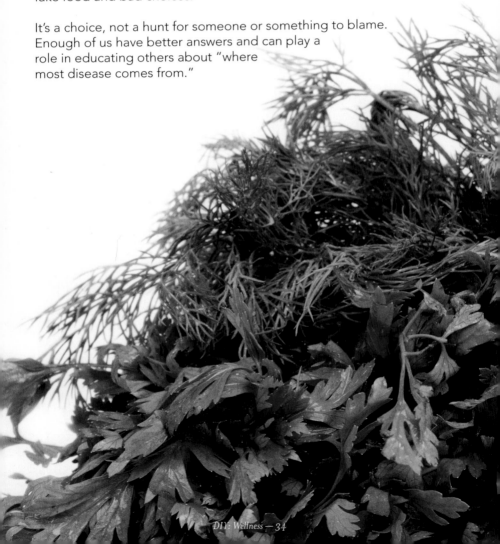

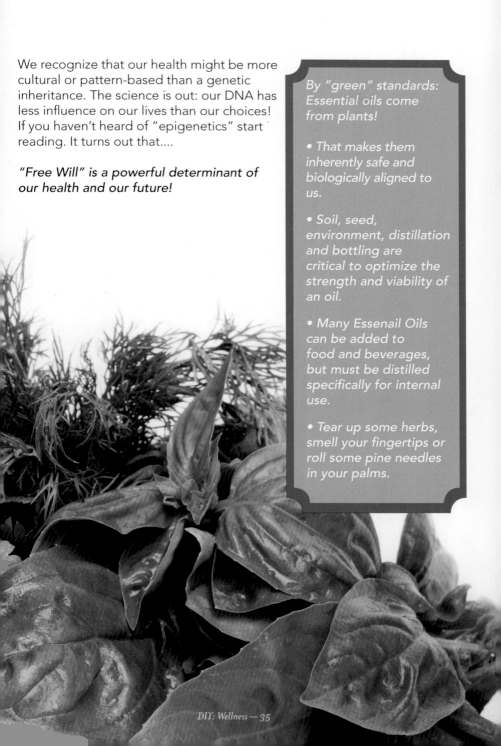

We recognize that our health might be more cultural or pattern-based than a genetic inheritance. The science is out: our DNA has less influence on our lives than our choices! If you haven't heard of "epigenetics" start reading. It turns out that....

"Free Will" is a powerful determinant of our health and our future!

By "green" standards: Essential oils come from plants!

• *That makes them inherently safe and biologically aligned to us.*

• *Soil, seed, environment, distillation and bottling are critical to optimize the strength and viability of an oil.*

• *Many Essenail Oils can be added to food and beverages, but must be distilled specifically for internal use.*

• *Tear up some herbs, smell your fingertips or roll some pine needles in your palms.*

POWER LOSS & SUGAR

More addicting than cocaine and offered to each generation as a reward or token of love. What was once a special occasion to serve dessert, has now become breakfast, lunch, and dinner. Processed carbohydrates, sugar in any form, (with the exception of natural fruits), should be considered a dessert. Any meal that neglects to have optimum amounts of vegetables, proteins and healthy fats, does not qualify as a meal. Real food does not have an ingredient list, complex code or mystery label.

A 2015 study showed 50% of the U.S. population is pre-diabetic or diabetic and the numbers are rising. It is an epidemic and there is a cause for this effect. What it does to our brains and our bodies isn't pretty, safe or affordable.

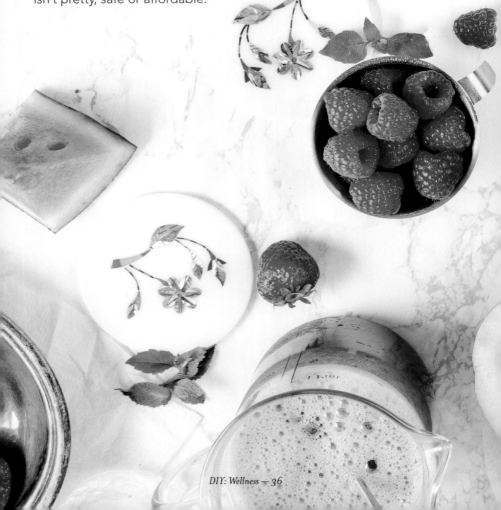

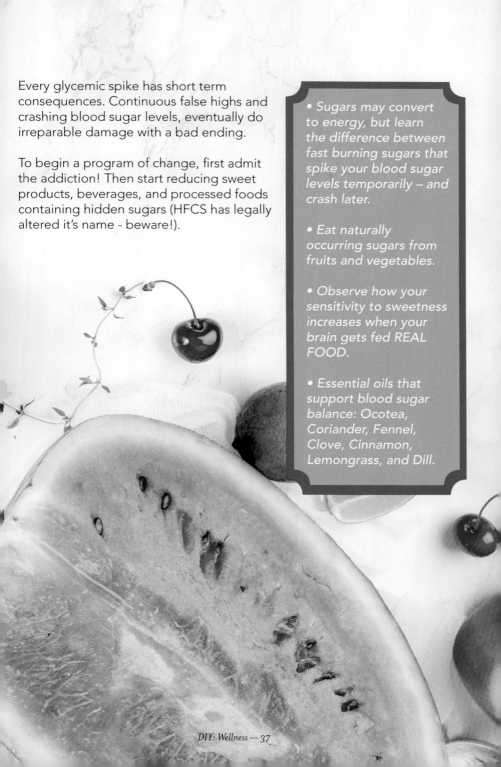

Every glycemic spike has short term consequences. Continuous false highs and crashing blood sugar levels, eventually do irreparable damage with a bad ending.

To begin a program of change, first admit the addiction! Then start reducing sweet products, beverages, and processed foods containing hidden sugars (HFCS has legally altered it's name - beware!).

- Sugars may convert to energy, but learn the difference between fast burning sugars that spike your blood sugar levels temporarily – and crash later.

- Eat naturally occurring sugars from fruits and vegetables.

- Observe how your sensitivity to sweetness increases when your brain gets fed REAL FOOD.

- Essential oils that support blood sugar balance: Ocotea, Coriander, Fennel, Clove, Cinnamon, Lemongrass, and Dill.

• Essential Oils help oxygenate the cells and raise our vibrational frequency.

• Avoid exposure to electronic things and environments that zap your energy.

• Make a habit of "oils in your pocket" wherever you go.

Wear a diffuser necklace and inhale an oil if you feel drained of energy in a high EMF room.

Top helpers: Frankincense, Cedarwood, Black Pepper, Sage, Peppermint.

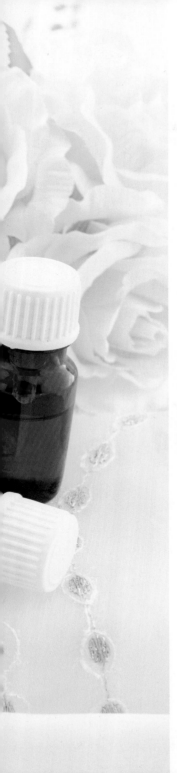

ZAPPED BY EMFs

Electro-magnetic fields are caused by 'stray voltage.' Electricity that has an excess of power that has not been used or rerouted and has no place to go.... goes under ground, across waterways, through your walls, from your electronic devices and into your body. In some European nations, it is considered a Class II carcinogen.

To reduce EMF toxicity, use filters designed to reduce stray voltage and protect you from computers, monitors, WiFi, cell phones, etc. You can find devices that will work in your home, schools, and offices to reduce EMFs.

If you have a limited budget, you can use sheets of aluminum foil to stand on, take baths with Epsom salts and increase your mineral intake since they help "ground" us.

Go barefoot outside as often as possible. The earth is highly charged with negative ions and a magnetic field that "grounds" us. It is highly charged after lightening storms.... wait 'til it's safe, go out barefooted and "feel it!"

And use essential oils! They all carry a vibrational frequency that our bodies absorb to help naturally enlighten us as well as ground us!

TOXIC OVERLOAD

At no other time in history (that we know of), have there been man-made chemicals unleashed in such great quantity or used without clear foresight of their potential harm to humans, animals, birds, bees, fish, air, water, or the earth. Every when new evidence points to stopping or restricting an industry from doing any more harm, it gets tied up in bureaucracy for so long, people forget "nothing has changed."

We are poisoning the earth and therefore.... our lives. Who do we think it ultimately responsible for our health, the lives of others, or the future of the planet? As 'consumers' we still have more power than we are led to believe!

Let's start at home with the choices that we make.

Things we can do now:
- Have your water tested
- Install good water filters
- Check for lead in pipes
- Read labels and ask questions
- Avoid chemical laden products, synthetic dyes and fragrances
- Use natural-based products
- Choose reusable containers
- Avoid plastic and nonstick pans
- Eat fresh, organic food
- Limit canned, processed junk
- Grow your own food
- Diffuser essential oils
- Educate yourself and others
- Advocate for change

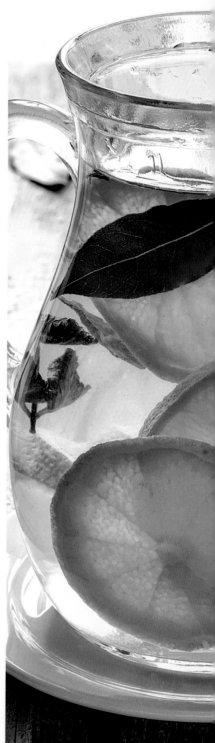

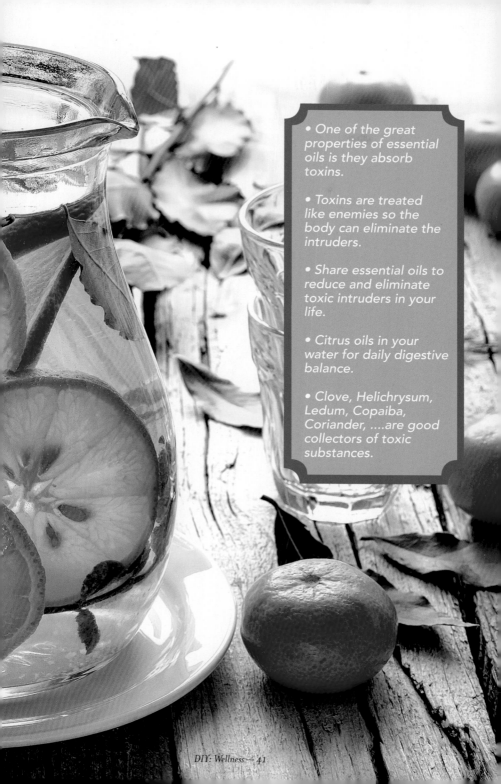

• One of the great properties of essential oils is they absorb toxins.

• Toxins are treated like enemies so the body can eliminate the intruders.

• Share essential oils to reduce and eliminate toxic intruders in your life.

• Citrus oils in your water for daily digestive balance.

• Clove, Helichrysum, Ledum, Copaiba, Coriander, ...are good collectors of toxic substances.

PARASITES OVERLOOKED

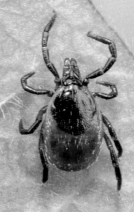

Contrary to the beliefs of conventional medicine in America, we do have critters. Lots of them. Most are harmless and we are capable of managing them with proper diets, strong immune systems, and by washing our food. Since we have a global distribution of food items now, parasites can become problematic.

Parasites can be the cause of a digestive complaint. A cheap stool sample could be tested, prior to more invasive and expensive procedures if mystery symptoms can't be easily traced.

If left undetected or misdiagnosed, you can spend thousands of dollars and months of frustration trying to understand your symptoms, if they fall into the category of "we don't know." Even Lyme Disease tests with negative results, can throw you off the path to resolution. Ask to be retested for less time and money than it takes "to wonder what's wrong" for six months or years of doctor visits.

Millions of people travel around the world now with easy access to remote adventures, humanitarian work and commerce. We are all subject to being exposed to rare and invasive critters. Our immune system has adaptive principals, but that takes time to strengthen against things that are foreign to our bodies.

Yes, there are parasites in the world....
and in America.

Fecal tests are inexpensive, but you have to request them nowadays. Keeping a healthy 'microbiome' and immune system is the best defense against most invasive critters.

- *Essential Oils protect plants from insects and parasites as a natural defense against invaders.*

- *Plants produce chemical compounds to defend their lives.*

- *One odor may attract a pollinator, while another one repels an invader.*

- *These characteristics can be passed on to help human beings.*

- *Copaiba, Lemongrass, Idaho Tansy, Anise, Ocotea, Peppermint, Tarragon....*

KEY CHANGES WITHIN

Good gut flora is one of the best markers of a healthy body. If we keep it in balance, it acts like a manager for every other system. As the saying goes, "garbage in, garbage out." We are responsible for maintaining our digestive system by the food choices and product choices we make. Remember: everything we breathe, everything we put on our skin, and everything we eat and drink, become part of us.

Our digestive system should be clean and efficient in its function to eliminate waste within 24 hours. Constipation and diarrhea are a sign that something's wrong. Our thoughts and behaviors are also being influenced by the junk inside us! Our entire digestive system and our liver are supposed to filter anything that is not natural to the human body and will impede our minds. Since bad fats don't allow for the release of toxins, eliminate them.

Due to the poor quality of our soil, our water, our food and mass production agricultural system, we need to supplement with minerals, enzymes and probiotics. We know that it is increasingly difficult to navigate these challenging times.

The mind, body and spirit require that we pay attention.

1. Are you taking care of and strengthening your emotional health?

2. Are you expressing your feelings in a healthy way?

3. Do you fill your heart with positive messages to balance the chatter in your brain?

4. Do you take time to meditate, pray, stretch or just sit with your thoughts?

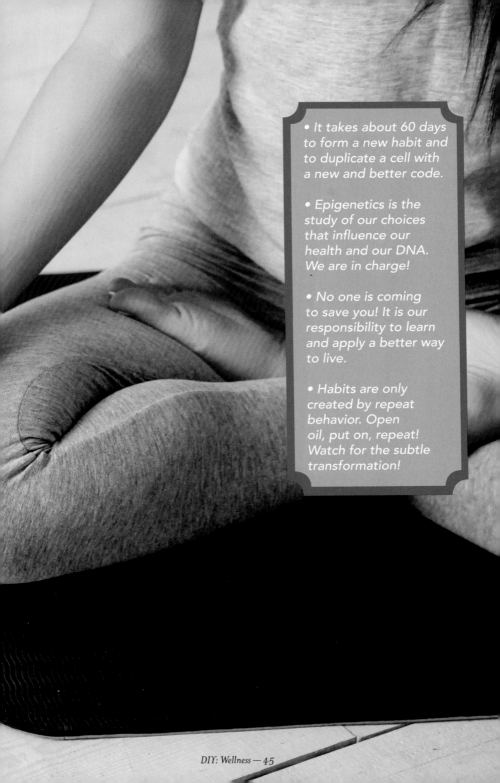

• It takes about 60 days to form a new habit and to duplicate a cell with a new and better code.

• Epigenetics is the study of our choices that influence our health and our DNA. We are in charge!

• No one is coming to save you! It is our responsibility to learn and apply a better way to live.

• Habits are only created by repeat behavior. Open oil, put on, repeat! Watch for the subtle transformation!

STRESS 101

The number one influence on our
emotional health - is stress. Why save
it for the end? Because in the end, it is
a primary cause of our failing health.
And in the end, we need to think long
and hard about our lifestyle choices and
who we surround ourselves with that
support our Higher Self, Our Purpose,
and Potential. Find good people! And
be one of them!

Good stress is "the element of activity
going on in our minds and bodies that
helps us create and evolve." Bad stress
paralyzes our activity (fight/flight) and
desire to move forward or contribute.
Bad stress also effects our digestive
system and creates an imbalance of
acid in the stomach, which decreases
the chance of nutrients reaching our
brains, nerves, blood, organs, muscles,
and bones. Learn to identify good
stress from bad.

Prolonged stress interferes with the
necessary nutrients reaching our body.
Stress can be a formula for fatigue,
illness, and despair. Technology has not
fulfilled the promise of a stress-free life.
It has created a new addiction. Love,
joy, peace, and play time might be a
cheaper and better device.

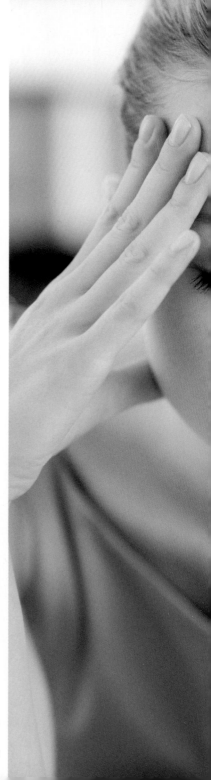

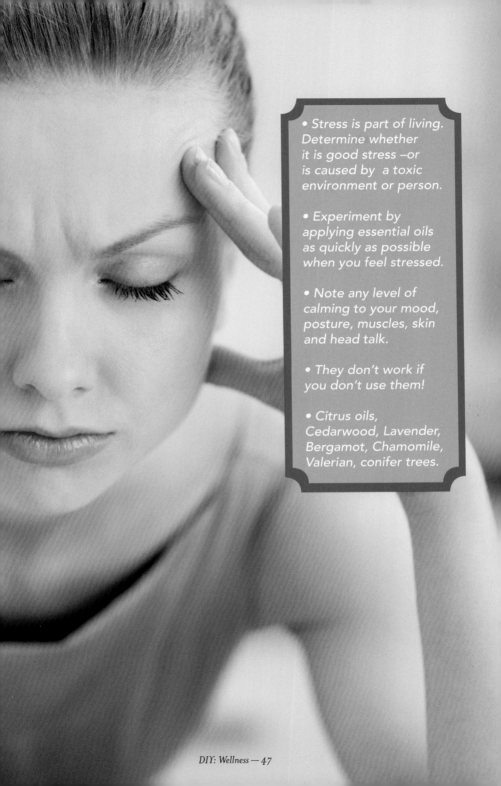

- Stress is part of living. Determine whether it is good stress —or is caused by a toxic environment or person.

- Experiment by applying essential oils as quickly as possible when you feel stressed.

- Note any level of calming to your mood, posture, muscles, skin and head talk.

- They don't work if you don't use them!

- Citrus oils, Cedarwood, Lavender, Bergamot, Chamomile, Valerian, conifer trees.

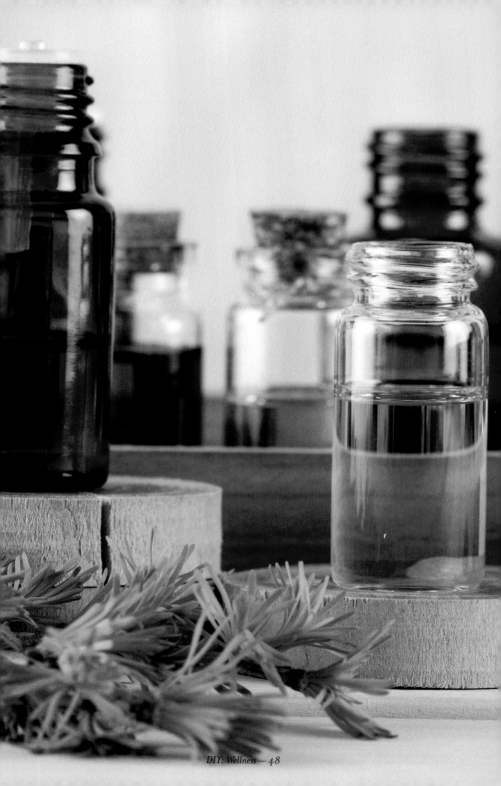

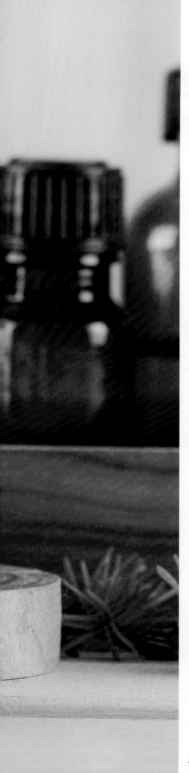

THE LIGHT WITHIN

Essential oils are used as a primary and first choice to "beat the blues," because of the power Aromatherapy has in connecting four of our five senses. Though our sense of smell gets less recognition than vision, hearing, touch and taste, it has the deepest connection to our memories and emotions. Our sense of smell integrates all the other senses, except for hearing. (Plants can't talk.)

We can see the trees, the leaves, the garden and the flowers. We can touch the flowers, the skin and the essential oil. We can taste the food, the herbs and feel the vital essence of the sun. Aromas inspire and create thoughts at the deepest level!

Since we have gradually lost touch with much that nature has to offer, we can restore the influence that it has on our happiness and well being. Bringing the outdoors in with essentials oils can shift our mood, lighten our hearts, and reconnect all our senses to a relationship with nature.

Essential oils are the essential essence of life. Each drop holds the life code of a plant: nature's code, the light of the sun and an ability to transfer the spectrum of light like a rainbow into our homes, our minds, our bodies, and our spirits.

3 SIMPLE WAYS TO USE ESSENTIAL OILS

1) Diffusing and Inhalation

Diffusing forces the oils into a larger space, and accomplishes more cleansing of the surrounding area than just personal inhaling. Diffusing actually works by dispersing the anti-microbial function of the oils. Inhaling the oils directly from an open bottle or in the palms of your hands, can quickly calm or elevate the senses for positive effects in the emotional and physical body, but doesn't effect a room that may harbor viruses, bacteria, molds, and fungus. Inhaling is the intimate action, used to reach the limbic system of your brain.

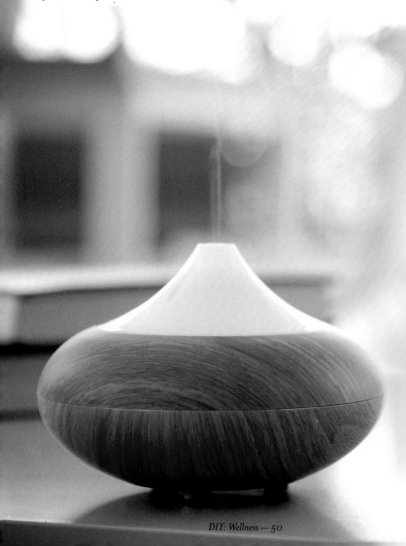

2) Topical Application
Placing a few drops of an essential oil in your hands or directly on the skin "neat" or "diluted," allowing the oils to penetrate the dermis within minutes to reach the cellular level of the body.

The feet are a safe first choice! They have the largest pores in the body. They are connected to every system in the body. They come in a variety of shapes, sizes, and colors and are really fun to play with!

It is advisable to dilute essential oils to extend coverage, prevent skin irritation, and limit evaporation. Use a well balanced massage oil, organic almond, jojoba, avocado, or unscented lotion. Every oil is unique and every 'body' is, too! Be willing to experiment, but follow safety precautions. Address any reactions by analyzing your diet. Learn to recognize – "what caused the effect!"

3) Internal Use
Please review current and cautionary viewpoints for internal use. Due to the unregulated guidelines for essential oils (GRAS: Generally Regarded As Safe) in the food industry, there are "essential oils" crossing over from the perfume industry that are not safe for internal use. Food grade essential oils may be used in cooking, but they should not be confused with therapeutic-grade oils that benefit our health, through natural, biological links that are in harmony with our bodies.

REFERENCES

Our introductory books are all compliant, compatible, and easy to use for your events and workshops:

Beat the Blues DIY: Keys to Wellness
Beauty and Body Care: DIY Naturally
DIY: Beauty
DIY: Lifestyle
Essential Oils R 4 U
Heart Scents
Barefoot and Sp'Oiled

by Star Moree & Kari McDermott

Feel free to Google search any of these wellness topics for more information.

"So many people spend their health gaining wealth.... Then have to spend their wealth to regain their health."

— A. J Reb Materi

We hope this little bit of information is like handing you a key to find your own answers and guide you toward a life of Wellness. Once you conquer the Wellness portion, you can pursue your Purpose, and when you are thriving and enjoying the work you love, Abundance is guaranteed!

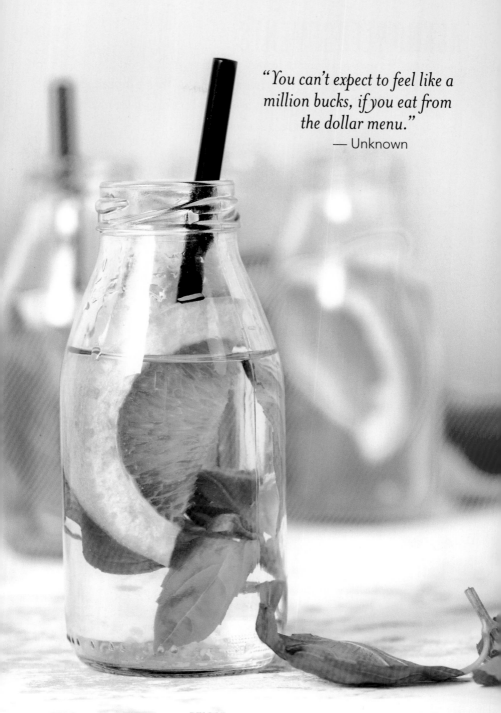

"You can't expect to feel like a million bucks, if you eat from the dollar menu."
— Unknown

ACKNOWLEDGEMENTS

Thank you for sharing this journey toward Wellness. We are proud to be part of every passionate team and person, whose life has changed because of Young Living's amazing products and continuous research.

There are millions of people waking up and taking responsibility for their choices, instead of finding excuses or denying their mysterious health problems and fatigue.

A book called DIY: Wellness, means you have to do it yourself at some level, but it's nice to have a little guidance on how to simply begin.

When we collectively begin to make choices that affect our bodies and the earth that sustains us…. the world's business practices and values will align to our intentions and our desires. Young Living already does!

Star Moree and Kari McDermott

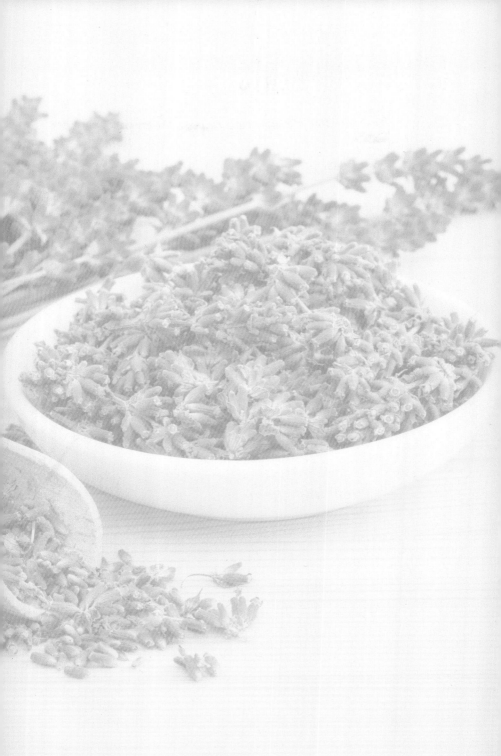